GW00481889

The Complete Keto Diet Cookies Collection for Beginners

Lose Weight and Enjoy this Big Collection of Delicious Keto Diet Cookies

Jessica Simpson

Contents

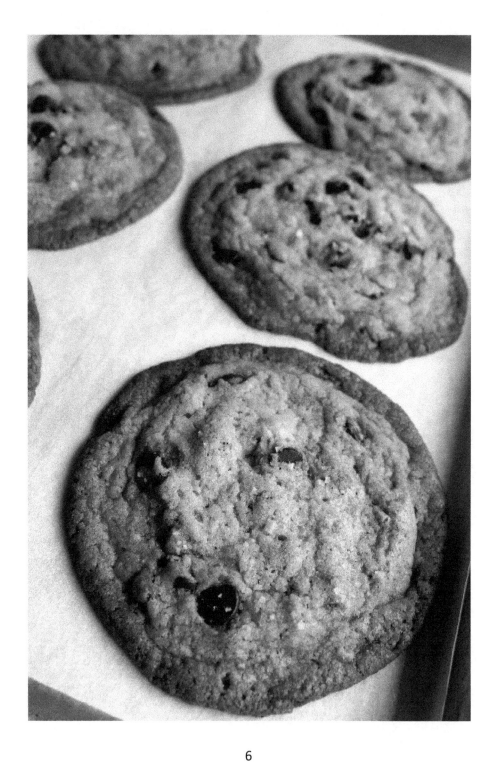

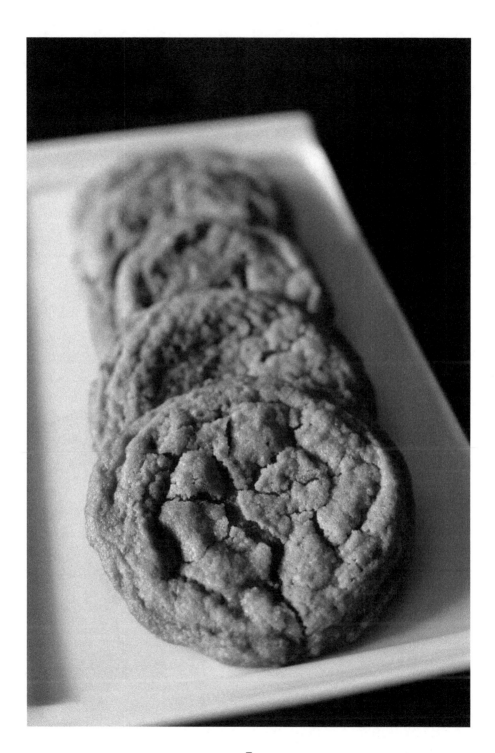

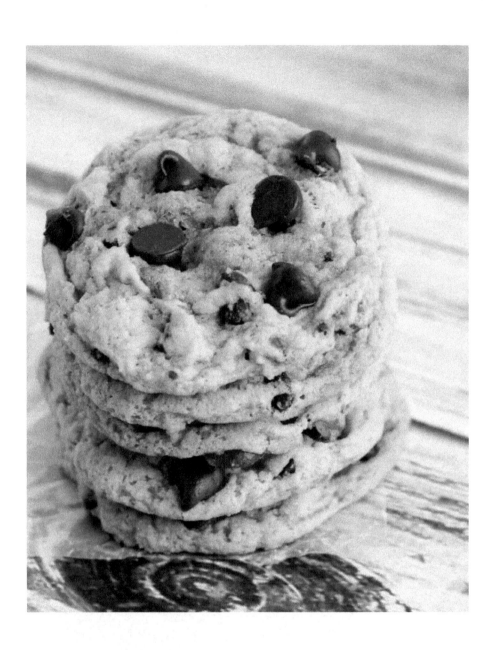

Chocolate Brownie

Servings: 6

Cooking Time: 25 Minutes

Ingredients:

- 1/4 cup almond flour1/3 cup monk fruit sweetener
- 2 tsp. cocoa powder, unsweetened
- 1/4 tsp. baking powder, gluten-free
- 2 tbsp. coconut oil
- 1 tsp. vanilla extract, sugar-free
- 4 oz. chocolate chips, sugar-free
- 1/4 cup pecans, chopped
- 1 large egg
- 1/4 tsp. salt

Directions:

1. Set your stove to 370° Fahrenheit. Set out a non-stick baking mat or cover a regular sized cookie sheet with baking paper.
2. Heat a saucepan to melt the chocolate chips and coconut oil until smooth.
3. In a regular dish, whip the sweetener and eggs until together.
4. Stir in the baking powder, vanilla extract and salt thoroughly.Pour the melted chocolate into the batter.

5. Add the almond flour and stir with a large spoon for about 1 minute. The dough will have a runny consistency.

6. Carefully stir the pecans and cocoa powder into the dough until fully incorporated.

7. Use a cookie scoop to spoon out 6 cookies onto the prepared baking sheet, placing the cookies about 2 inches apart.

8. Heat for 10 – 12 minutes and move to the counter. Wait approximately 20 minutes before serving.

9. Tricks and Tips:

10. If you prefer a brownie texture to the cookies, take the baking sheet out of the stove after 12 minutes.

11. If you would like the taste of the cookies to have more chocolate flavor, add an additional 1/4 cup of chocolate chips when you fold the pecans into the batter.

Nutrition Info: 2 grams ;Net Carbs: 1.3 grams ;Fat: 8 grams ;Calories:

Easy No Bake Cookies

Servings: 20

Cooking Time: 5 Minutes

Ingredients:

- 1 tsp swerve
- 2 tbsp butter, melted
- 2 cups unsweetened coconut flakes
- 2 tbsp unsweetened cocoa powder
- 1 ½ tsp vanilla
- 1 13 cup peanut butter, creamy

Directions:

1. Line baking tray with parchment paper and set aside.
2. Add all ingredients into the large bowl and mix until well combined.
3. Scoop batter onto a baking tray and using back of spoon press dough down gently to make a cookie shape.
4. Place in refrigerator for 30 minutes.
5. Serve and enjoy.

Nutrition Info: Per Servings: Net Carbs: 3.4g; Calories: 18 Total Fat: 16.3g; Saturated Fat: 8.2g Protein: 5.2g; Carbs: 6.2g; Fiber: 2.8g; Sugar: 2.5g; Fat 80% Protein 12% Carbs 8%

Fudgy Brownie Cookies

Servings: 12

Cooking Time: 12 Minutes

Ingredients:

- 2 tbsp butter, softened
- 1 egg, room temperature
- 1 tbsp Truvia
- ¼ cup Swerve
- 1/8 tsp blackstrap molasses
- 1 tbsp VitaFiber syrup
- 1 tsp vanilla extract
- 6 tbsp sugar-free chocolate chips
- 1 tsp butter
- 6 tbsp almond flour
- 1 tbsp cocoa powder
- 1/8 tsp baking powder
- 1/8 tsp salt
- ¼ tsp xanthan gum
- ¼ cup chopped pecans
- 1 tbsp sugar-free chocolate chips

Directions:

1. Beat egg with 2 tablespoons butter, VitaFiber, sweeteners, and vanilla in a bowl with a hand mixer.

2. Melt ½ of a tablespoon of the chocolate chips with 1 teaspoon of butter in a bowl by heating them in the microwave for 30 seconds then stir well.
3. Add this mixture to the first butter mixture and mix well until smooth.
4. Stir in all the dry ingredients and mix until smooth.
5. Fold in remaining chocolate chips and pecans.
6. Place this batter in the freezer for 8 minutes.
7. Let your oven preheat at 350 degrees F.
8. Grease a baking sheet and drop batter scoop by scoop onto it to form small cookies.
9. Flatten the cookies lightly then bake for 10 minutes.
10. Allow the cookies to cool for about 15 minutes then serve.

Nutrition Info: Calories 288 Total Fat 25.3 g Saturated Fat 6.7 g Cholesterol 23 mg Sodium 74 mg Total Carbs 9.6 g Sugar 0.1 g Fiber 3.8 g Protein 7.6 g

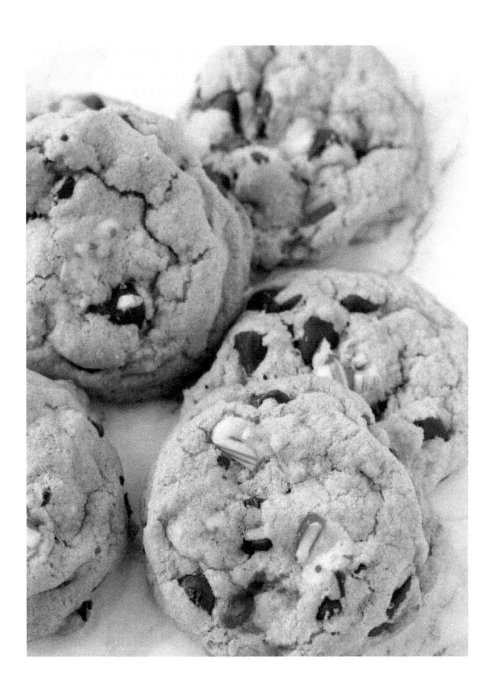

Peppermint Chocolate Cookies

Servings: 30

Cooking Time: 40 Minutes

Ingredients:

- 1 1/2 cup almond flour
- 1/4 cup coconut flour
- 1 cup mixed chocolate chips, divided
- 2 tablespoons cocoa powder
- 1/8 teaspoon sea salt
- 2 tablespoons erythritol sweetener
- 1/4 cup monk fruit sweetener
- 1 scoop chocolate protein powder
- 1/2 teaspoon peppermint extract, unsweetened
- 1/2 cup cashew butter
- Coconut milk as needed

Directions:

1. Place flours in a large bowl, add cocoa powder, salt, sweetener, and protein powder and stir well, set aside until required.
2. Place butter in a heatproof bowl, add monk fruit sweetener and microwave for 45 seconds or until butter is melt.
3. Stir well until combined, then stir in mint extract and add to flour mixture.

4. Mix well until crumbly batter comes together and then slowly stir in milk until thick batter comes together.

5. Fold in half of the chocolate chips, then shape mixture into small cookie balls and place on a cookie sheet lined with parchment paper.

6. Press each cookie ball slightly, top with remaining chocolate chips and refrigerate for 30 minutes or more until firm.

7. Serve straightaway.

Nutrition Info: Calories: Cal, Carbs: 4.4 g, Fat: 7 g, Protein: 2.2 g, Fiber: 2 g.

Double-chocolate Keto Cookies

Servings: 8

Cooking Time: 12 Minutes

Ingredients:

- ¾ cup 2 tablespoons almond flour
- 1 tablespoon gelatine, grass-fed
- ½ teaspoon baking soda
- ½ teaspoon salt
- ¼ cup butter, unsalted, softened
- 3 tablespoons cocoa powder
- ½ teaspoon vanilla essence
- ¼ cup almond butter
- ½ cup granulated erythritol
- 1 large egg, room temperature
- ⅓ cup sugar free dark-chocolate, diced

Directions:

1. Let your oven preheat at 350 degrees F. layer 2 baking trays with wax paper.
2. Mix almond flour with gelatin, baking soda, salt and cocoa powder in a suitable bowl.
3. Beat butter with sweetener and almond butter in an electric mixer.
4. Add egg and vanilla while beating the mixture.

5. Stir in almond flour mixture and mix well to form a dough.

6. Fold chocolate chunks then make 1-inch balls out of it.

7. Place these balls in the baking trays.

8. Press each ball into ½ inch thick cookie.

9. Bake these cookies for 12 minutes.

10. Allow them to cool at room temperature.

11. Serve.

Nutrition Info: Per Servings: Calories 198 Total Fat 19.2 g Saturated Fat 11.5 g Cholesterol mg Total Carbs 4.5 g Sugar 3.3 g Fiber 0.3 g Sodium 142 mg Potassium 34 mg Protein 3.4 g

Pine Nut Cookies

Servings: 20

Cooking Time: 12 Minutes

Ingredients:

- 1 Large egg
- 1 Teaspoon of almond extract
- 1 Pinch of salt
- 1 Cup of stevia
- 2 Cups of superfine blanched almond flour
- 1/3 Cup of pine nuts

Directions:

1. Preheat your oven to a temperature of about 325 degrees Fahrenheit.
2. Mix the eggs with the almond extract, the salt and the sweetener in a bowl of a medium.
3. Beat your ingredients with a mixer for about 2 minutes or until the mixture becomes glossy.
4. Add in the almond flour and beat your ingredients until it becomes fluffy.
5. If the dough gets too dry, add about tablespoon of water in a way that it holds up very well together.
6. Place the nuts over a small platter.
7. Take a pinch of the dough and roll it into one piece of about 1 inch in its diameter.

8. Press the top of the ball dough into the nut with the side up.

9. Place the cookie over a parchment paper lined cookie sheet lined with a parchment paper.

10. Repeat the same process with the remaining dough; you can get about 20 cookies.

11. Bake your cookies in the oven for about 12 minutes.

12. Remove the cookies from the oven and let cool for about 6 minutes.

13. Serve and enjoy your cookies.

Nutrition Info: Calories: 83;Fat: 7.5 g;Carbohydrates: 2.4g;Fiber: 1g;Protein: 4 g

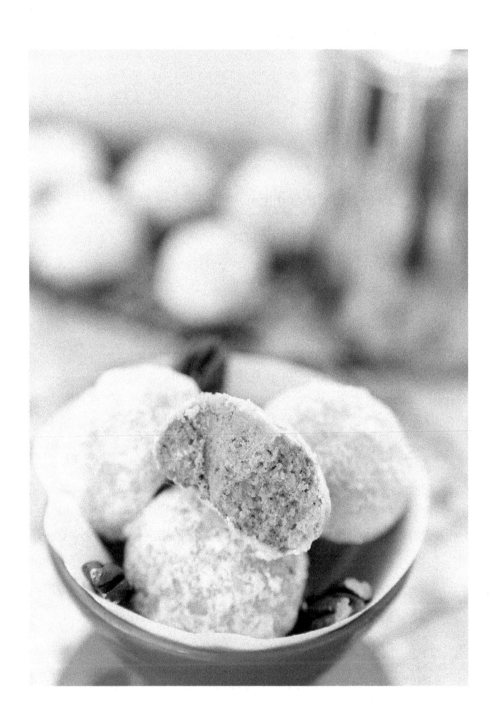

Pecan Snowball Cookies

Servings: 8

Cooking Time: 15 Minutes

Ingredients:

- 8 tbsp butter
- 1 1/2 cup almond flour
- 1 cup pecans, chopped
- 1/2 cup Swerve
- 1 tsp vanilla essence
- 1/2 tsp vanilla liquid stevia
- 1/4 tsp salt
- extra confectioners to roll balls in

Directions:

1. Let your oven preheat at 350 degrees F.
2. Put all the dough ingredients in a food processor and blend well to form a dough ball.
3. Layer a baking sheet with parchment paper.
4. Add cookie batter to the baking sheet scoop by scoop to make 2separate mounds.
5. Spread these mounds into flat cookies.
6. Freeze them for 30 minutes then bake them for 15 minutes.
7. Allow them to cool then roll the cookies in the swerve confectioners.

8. Serve.

Nutrition Info: Per Servings: Calories 252 Total Fat 17.3 g Saturated Fat 11.5 g Cholesterol 141 mg Total Carbs 7.2 g Sugar 0.3 g Fiber 1.4 g Sodium 153 mg Potassium 73 mg Protein 5.2 g

Pistachio Muffins

Servings: 12

Cooking Time: 30 Minutes

Ingredients:

- 4 Large Eggs, it is better to use brown Eggs
- ½ Cup of almond butter, unsalted
- ¼ Cup of confectioners Swerve
- ¼ Cup of Organic Stevia Blend by Pyure
- 1 Teaspoon of Pistachio Extract
- ½ Cup of Almond Milk, unsweetened
- 1 Teaspoon of Vanilla Extract
- 1 Cup of blanched Almond Flour
- ½ Cup of Organic Coconut Flour
- 2 Teaspoons of Baking Powder
- ½ Teaspoon of Xanthan Gum
- 1 Teaspoon of Himalayan Pink Salt
- ½ Cup of crushed Pistachio Nuts

Directions:

1. Preheat your oven to about 325 F.
2. Whisk the eggs in a large mixing bowl until they becomes fluffy.
3. In a separate bowl, melt the almond butter until it becomes soft.

4. Add the butter to a bowl with the sweeteners, the extracts, and the almond milk.
5. Blend your ingredients until it is very well incorporated.
6. Add the Pistachio Extract, the vanilla Extract, the almond Flour, the coconut flour, the baking powder; the Xanthan gum and the salt.
7. Whisk your ingredients until they becomes very well mixed.
8. Add your dry ingredients into a large bowl and mix very we well.
9. Add the crushed pistachios; then fold until it is blended.
10. Grease a muffin tin of about 12 cups or liners.
11. Evenly pour the batter into each of the muffin cups.
12. Bake the muffins for about 25 to 30 minutes.
13. Let your muffins cool for about 5 minutes.
14. Serve and enjoy your muffins!

Nutrition Info: Calories: 198;Fat: 12 g;Carbohydrates: 11g;Fiber: 2g;Protein: 6

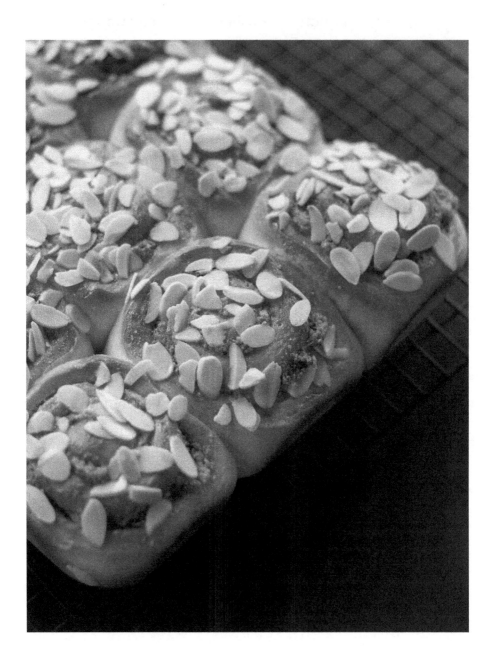

Almond Cinnamon Butter

Servings: 12

Cooking Time: 25 Minutes

Ingredients:

- 2 cups blanched almond flour
- 1 tsp. ground cinnamon
- 1/2 cup butter, softened
- 1 large egg
- 1/2 cup Swerve sweetener, granulated
- 1 tsp. vanilla extract, sugar-free

Directions:

1. Set the stove temperature at 350° Fahrenheit. Use a non-stick baking mat if available or layer baking paper on a regular sized cookie sheet.
2. In a big dish, whisk the almond flour and butter completely.
3. Combine the sweetener and egg making sure the mixture is not lumpy.Then add the vanilla extract and cinnamon until incorporated.Use a cookie scooper to spoon out a small amount and roll by hand into 1 inch balls. Transfer to the prepared cookie sheet.
4. Using a fork, press the cookies firmly, first horizontally and then vertically to create a crisscross pattern.

5. Heat for 12 - 1minutes in the stove. Remove and place on the counter to cool before serving.

Nutrition Info: 3 grams ;Net Carbs: 1.2 grams ;Fat: 13 grams ;Calories: 196

Cream Cheese

Servings: 15

Cooking Time: 1 Hour 25 Minutes

Ingredients:

- 1/2 cup coconut flour
- 1/4 tsp. salt
- 1/2 tsp. baking powder, gluten-free
- 3 tbsp. cream cheese, softened
- 1/2 cup Swerve sweetener, granulated
- 1 large egg
- 1/2 cup butter, softened
- 1 tsp. vanilla extract, sugar-free

Directions:

1. Place a piece of baking paper to the side.
2. In a big dish, cream the sweetener, vanilla extract and cream cheese with an electrical beater until smooth. Add the butter and egg and stir until incorporated.
3. Finally, mix the almond flour, baking powder and salt to the mixture, making sure the batter is not lumpy.
4. Transfer the dough to the piece of baking paper and mold into a log. Crimp the sides of the paper securely and harden in the refrigerator for approximately 60 minutes.Set the stove to the temperature of 350° Fahrenheit. Cover a regular sized cookie sheet with

baking paper. Alternatively, use a non-stick baking mat.

5. Remove the firmed dough from the refrigerator and slice into half inch pieces.

6. Place on the prepared flat pan with approximately 2 inches space in between and heat in the stove for 15 - 18 minutes. When the cookies are done, they will be brown on the edges.

7. Cool the cookies on the counter for at least 10 minutes before serving.

Nutrition Info: 1 gram ;Net Carbs: 1 gram ;Fat: grams ;Calories: 91

Buttery Energy Bites

Servings: 8

Cooking Time: 0 Minutes

Ingredients:

- 1 cup almond flour
- 3 tablespoons butter
- 2 tablespoons erythritol
- 1 teaspoon vanilla essence
- pinch of salt

Directions:

1. Put all the ingredients in a suitable bowl.
2. Whisk this mixture until well combined.
3. Divide the cookie dough into small cookies on a baking sheet.
4. Place the cookie/baking sheet in the refrigerator to chill for 1 hour.
5. Enjoy after bringing it to room temperature.

Nutrition Info: Calories 114 ;Total Fat 9.g ;Saturated Fat 4.5 g ;Cholesterol 10 mg ;Sodium 155 mg ;Total Carbs 3.1 g ;Sugar 1.4 g ;Fiber 1.5 g ;Protein 3.5 g

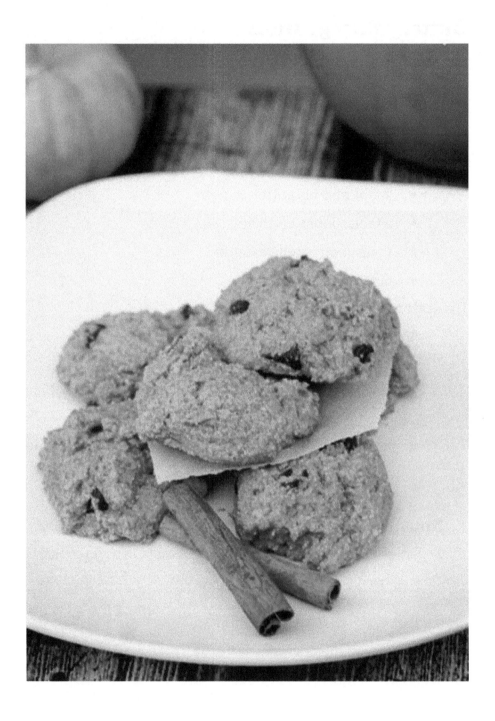

Pumpkin Butter Cookies

Servings: 8

Cooking Time: 25 Minutes

Ingredients:

- ¼ cup pumpkin puree
- 1 large egg
- 1 cup almond flour
- ½ tsp baking powder
- ½ tsp pumpkin pie spice
- ½ tsp vanilla essence
- ¼ cup butter
- ¼ cup powdered erythritol
- ¼ cup Lily's chocolate chips, dark

Directions:

1. Let your oven preheat at 350 degrees F.
2. Beat pumpkin puree with butter in an electric mixer.
3. Add egg, baking powder, vanilla essence, erythritol, and almond flour. Mix well.
4. Once smooth fold in chocolate chips and mix gently.
5. Divide this dough into equal size balls and flatten these balls into cookies.
6. Bake them for 25 minutes in the cookie tray until golden.
7. Allow them to cool then serve.

8. Enjoy.

Nutrition Info: Per Servings: Calories 1 Total Fat 14.3 g Saturated Fat 10.5 g Cholesterol 175 mg Total Carbs 4.5 g Sugar 0.5 g Fiber 0.3 g Sodium 125 mg Potassium 83 mg Protein 3.2 g

Peanut Butter

Servings: 10

Cooking Time: 20 Minutes

Ingredients:

- 1/2 cup peanut butter
- 1 large egg
- 1/2 cup Swerve sweetener, confectioners
- 1/2 tsp. vanilla extract, sugar-free

Directions:

1. Set your stove to the temperature of 350° Fahrenheit. Layer a regular sized cookie sheet with baking paper. You can also use a non-stick baking mat.
2. In a regular dish, blend the egg, Swerve, peanut butter and vanilla extract with a large rubber scraper.
3. Scoop out 1 1/2 tablespoons of dough with a spoon and roll into small balls. Place them on the prepared cookie sheet or mat.
4. Press the cookie balls with a fork, first horizontally and then vertically to create a crisscross pattern.
5. Heat in the stove for 12 - 1minutes and transfer to the counter.
6. Wait 10 minutes to serve and enjoy!
7. Tricks and Tips:

8. If you want an extra afternoon boost, add in a large scoop of protein powder into your peanut butter cookies.

Nutrition Info: 3 grams ;Net Carbs: 2.5 grams ;Fat: 6 grams ;Calories: 82

Cheese Coconut Cookies

Servings: 15

Cooking Time: 18 Minutes

Ingredients:

- 1 egg
- 12 cup butter, softened
- 3 tbsp cream cheese, softened
- 12 cup coconut flour
- 12 tsp baking powder
- 1 tsp vanilla
- 12 cup erythritol
- Pinch of salt

Directions:

1. In a bowl, whisk together butter, erythritol, and cream cheese.
2. Add egg and vanilla and beat until smooth and creamy.
3. Add coconut flour, salt, and baking powder and beat until well combined.
4. Place mixture into the bowl and cover with parchment paper.
5. Place in refrigerator for 1 hour.
6. Preheat the oven to 350 F 180 C.
7. Spray a baking tray with cooking spray.
8. Remove cookie dough from refrigerator.

9. Make cookies from dough and place onto a baking tray.

10. Bake for 15-18 minutes or until lightly golden brown.

11. Remove from oven and set aside to cool completely.

12. Serve and enjoy.

Nutrition Info: Per Servings: Net Carbs: 0.3g; Calories: 68; Total Fat: 7.2g; Saturated Fat: 4.5g Protein: 0.7g; Carbs: 0.5g; Fiber: 0.2g; Sugar: 0.1g; Fat 95% Protein 4% Carbs 1%

Gingersnap Cookies

Servings: 8

Cooking Time: 10 Minutes

Ingredients:

- 1 egg
- ½ tsp vanilla
- 18 tsp ground cloves
- ¼ tsp ground nutmeg
- ¼ tsp ground cinnamon
- ½ tsp ground ginger
- 1 tsp baking powder
- ¾ cup erythritol
- 24 cup butter, melted
- 1 ½ cups almond flour
- Pinch of salt

Directions:

1. In a mixing bowl, mix together all dry ingredients.
2. In another bowl, mix together all wet ingredients.
3. Add dry ingredients to the wet ingredients and mix until dough-like mixture is formed.
4. Cover and place in the refrigerator for 30 minutes.
5. Preheat the oven to 3 F 180 C.
6. Line baking tray with parchment paper and set aside.

7. Make cookies from dough and place on a prepared baking tray.

8. Bake in for 10-15 minutes.

9. Serve and enjoy.

Nutrition Info: Per Servings: Net Carbs: 2.8g; Calories: 232; Total Fat: 22.6g; Saturated Fat: 8.2g Protein: 5.3g; Carbs: 5.1g; Fiber: 2.3g; Sugar: 0.8g; Fat 87% Protein 9% Carbs 4%

Almond Butter Brownie Cookies

Servings: 6

Cooking Time: 12 Minutes

Ingredients:

- 1 cup almond butter
- 1/4 cup sugar free chocolate chips
- 1 large egg
- 4 tbsp sugar free cocoa powder
- 1/2 cup granulated erythritol
- 3 tbsp almond milk

Directions:

1. Let the oven preheat at 350 degrees F.
2. Combine almond butter, egg, cocoa powder and sweetener in a suitable bowl.
3. Add tbsp almond milk and mix well to make a soft dough.
4. Fold in chocolate chips then make small balls out of it.
5. Place these balls in the baking sheets and press them in thick cookies.
6. Bake these cookies for 12 minutes in the preheated oven.
7. Allow them to cool then serve.

Nutrition Info: Per Servings: Calories 2 Total Fat 25.3 g Saturated Fat 6.7 g Cholesterol 23 mg Total Carbs 9.6 g Sugar 0.1 g Fiber 3.8 g Sodium 74 mg Potassium 3 mg Protein 7.6 g

Stuffed Oreo Cookies

Servings: 8

Cooking Time: 12 Minutes

Ingredients:

- 1 1/3 cup almond flour
- 6 tbsp cocoa powder
- 2 tbsp black cocoa powder
- ¾ tsp kosher salt
- ½ tsp xanthan gum
- ½ tsp baking soda
- ¼ tsp espresso powder
- 5 ½ tbsp butter
- 8 tbsp erythritol
- 1 egg
- For Vanilla Cream Filling
- 4 tbsp grass-fed butter
- 1 tbsp coconut oil
- 1 ½ tsp vanilla extract
- Pinch kosher salt
- ½ - 1 cup Swerve confectioner sugar substitute

Directions:

1. Whisk almond flour, salt, both cocoa powders, xanthan gum, baking soda, and espresso powder in a suitable bowl.

2. Beat butter well in a large bowl with a hand mixer for minutes.
3. Whisk in sweetener and continue beating for 5 minutes then add the egg.
4. Beat well then add the flour mixture. Mix well until fully incorporated.
5. Wrap the cookie dough with plastic wrap and refrigerate for 1 hour.
6. Meanwhile, preheat your oven to 350 degrees F and layer a baking sheet with wax paper.
7. Place the dough in between two sheets of parchment paper.
8. Roll the dough out into a 1/inch thick sheet.
9. Cut 1 ¾ inch round cookies out of this sheet and reroll the dough to cut more cookies.
10. Spread these cookies on the baking sheet and freeze for 15 minutes.
11. Bake these cookies for 12 minutes then allow them to cool on a wire rack.
12. Beat butter with coconut oil in a bowl with an electric mixer.
13. Stir in vanilla extract, powdered sweetener to taste, and a pinch of salt.
14. Mix well then transfer it to a piping bag.
15. Place half of the cookies on a cookie sheet and top them with the cream filling.

16. Place the remaining half of the cookies over the filling to cover it.

17. Refrigerate for 15 minutes then serve.

Nutrition Info: Calories 215 Total Fat 20 g Saturated Fat 7 g Cholesterol 38 mg Sodium 12 mg Total Carbs 8 g Sugar 1 g Fiber 6 g Protein 5 g

Peanut Butter Cookies

Servings: 4

Cooking Time: 40 Minutes

Ingredients:

- 6 tablespoons coconut flour
- 2 tablespoon chocolate chips, unsweetened
- 1 tablespoon monk fruit sweetener
- ¾ cup peanut butter

Directions:

1. Place butter in a bowl, add sweetener and stir well until mixed.
2. Then add coconut flour and stir well until thick dough comes together, add more flour if the batter is too thin or more liquid if the batter is too thick.
3. Shape dough into four balls and place on a plate, lined with parchment paper.
4. Press cookie balls lightly, top with chocolate chips and place into refrigerator for 30 minutes or until firm.
5. Serve straightaway.

Nutrition Info: Calories: 282 Cal, Carbs: g, Fat: 21 g, Protein: 19 g, Fiber: 4 g.

Crispy Butter Cookies

Servings: 24

Cooking Time: 15 Minutes

Ingredients:

- 1 egg, lightly beaten
- 1 tsp vanilla
- 1 tsp baking powder
- 1 stick butter
- ¾ cup Swerve
- 1 ¼ cups almond flour
- Pinch of salt

Directions:

1. In a bowl, beat butter and sweetener until creamy.
2. In another bowl, mix together almond flour and baking powder.
3. Add egg and vanilla in butter mixture and beat until smooth.
4. Add dry ingredients to the wet ingredients and mix until well combined.
5. Wrap dough in plastic wrap and place in the fridge for 1 hour.
6. Preheat the oven 325 F 1 C.
7. Line baking tray with parchment paper and set aside.

8. Make cookies from dough and place on a prepared baking tray.

9. Bake for 15 minutes.

10. Allow to cool completely then serve.

Nutrition Info: Per Servings: Net Carbs: 0.8g; Calories: 71 Total Fat: 6.9g; Saturated Fat: 2.7g Protein: 1.5g; Carbs: 1.4g; Fiber: 0.6g; Sugar: 0.2g; Fat 87% Protein 8% Carbs 5%

Low-carb Coconut Shortbread Cookies

Servings: 8

Cooking Time: 12 Minutes

Ingredients:

- 3 tablespoons butter, melted
- ¼ cup confectioners' powdered erythritol
- 3 tablespoons finely shredded coconut, unsweetened
- 1 cup superfine blanched almond flour
- ½ teaspoon coconut extract

Directions:

1. Add butter, sweetener, flour and coconut extract into a bowl and mix well using a fork until well incorporated.
2. Bring together the dough and roll into a log of about 4 inches in length, using your palms.
3. Place over a sheet of cling wrap and wrap it tightly.
4. Unwrap and scatter coconut all over the dough.
5. Wrap the dough back up tightly. Freeze for 30 to 40 minutes.
6. Remove from the freezer and place on your cutting board. Remove the cling wrap and cut into ½ inch thick pieces.
7. Place on a baking sheet lined with parchment paper.

8. Bake in a preheated oven at 350° F for about 12-15 minutes or until golden brown.

9. Remove the baking sheet from the oven and let the cookies cool completely on the baking sheet.

10. Transfer into an airtight container. These can keep for 5-6 days at room temperature. If you freeze the cookies these can keep for 3 months.

Nutrition Info: per Servings: Calories: 131.3 kcal, Fat: 12.3 g, Carbohydrates: 4.1 g, Protein: 3.1 g

Mint Cream Keto Cookies

Servings: 22

Cooking Time: 18 Minutes

Ingredients:

- 4 ounces cream cheese, softened
- ½ cup + 2 tablespoons Swerve granular sweetener
- 1 egg
- ¼ teaspoon peppermint extract
- 1 teaspoon baking powder
- Few drops green food coloring
- Few drops red food coloring
- ¼ cup butter, at room temperature
- ¼ teaspoon xanthan gum
- ½ teaspoon vanilla extract
- 1 ¼ cups almond flour
- 1/8 teaspoon sea salt

Directions:

1. Line a large cookie sheet with parchment paper.
2. Add almond flour, xanthan gum, salt and baking powder into a large bowl. Mix well.
3. Add butter and cream cheese into a mixing bowl. Beat with an electric mixer at medium- high speed until it turns creamy. Beat in the sweetener.

4. Add egg, peppermint and vanilla extracts and beat well.

5. Lower the speed to low. Add the flour mixture and beat until just combined. Do not overbeat.

6. Make 3 equal portions of the dough and place each portion in a bowl.

7. Add a few drops red food coloring in one bowl. Add a few drops green food coloring into the 2nd bowl. Leave the dough in the 3rd bowl as it is.

8. Mix green color in 1st bowl and red color in the 2nd bowl.

9. Place the bowls in the refrigerator for at least an hour.

10. Remove the bowls from the refrigerator and place on your countertop.

11. To make a cookie: Take 1 teaspoon of dough from each of the 3 bowls. Bring them together and shape into a ball. Place on the prepared baking sheet. Press it lightly if desired or let it have the shape of a ball.

12. Repeat the previous step and make the remaining cookies. Leave some gap between the cookies while placing on the baking sheet.

13. Bake in a preheated oven at 325° F for about 18 to 20 minutes. They will appear less cooked. Do not bake for too long.

14. Remove from the oven and cool for 15 minutes. Remove the cookies carefully with a metal spatula and cool on a wire rack.

15. Cool completely. These cookies will be soft in texture.

16. Transfer into an airtight container. Refrigerate until use. These can keep for 2 weeks. If you freeze the cookies they can keep for 3 months.

Nutrition Info: per Servings: Calories: kcal, Fat: 16.9 g, Carbohydrates: 4 g, Protein: 4 g

Chocolate Chip

Servings: 12

Cooking Time: 25 Minutes

Ingredients:

- 1/2 tsp. apple cider vinegar1/4 tsp. Stevia sweetener, confectioner
- 1/2 tsp. baking soda
- 1 cup butter, cashew
- 2 large eggs
- 1 cup chocolate chips, stevia-sweetened
- 1/2 tsp. vanilla extract, sugar-free

Directions:

1. Set the stove to heat at 350° Fahrenheit. Use a non-stick baking mat or line a regular sized cooking sheet with baking paper.
2. In a food processor on the medium setting, whip the eggs until smooth. Add the sweetener and baking soda until mixed.
3. Add the apple cider vinegar and vanilla extract and stir with a rubber scraper.Finally, combine the butter to the batter and mix completely.
4. Use a cookie scooper to spoon the dough to the prepared flat pan approximately 2 inches away from each other.

5. Heat in the stove for 12 – 14 minutes and transfer the cookies to the counter for 10 minutes to cool before serving.

Nutrition Info: 5 grams ;Net Carbs: 10 grams ;Fat: 14 grams ;Calories: 178

Sesame Keto Bread

Servings: 8

Cooking Time: 60 Minutes

Ingredients:

- 5 tbsp ground psyllium husk powder
- 1¼ cup almond flour
- 2 tsp baking powder
- 1 tsp sea salt
- 1 cup water
- 2 tsp cider vinegar
- 3 egg whites
- 2 tbsp sesame seeds (optional)

Directions:

1. Preheat your oven to 350 degrees F.
2. Pour water in a pot then boil it.
3. Meanwhile, mix the dry ingredients for the batter in a suitable bowl.
4. Beat egg whites and vinegar in a separate bowl then stir in boiled water and dry mixture.
5. Beat it for 30 seconds with a hand mixer until smooth.
6. Make six rolls out of this dough then place them on a greased baking sheet.
7. Sprinkle sesame seeds over the rolls and press them gently.

8. Bake them for 60 minutes on the lower rack and garnish as desired.

9. Enjoy.

Nutrition Info: Calories 151 Total Fat 12.2 g Saturated Fat 2.4 g Cholesterol 1mg Sodium 276 mg Total Carbs 3.2 g Fiber 1.9 g Sugar 0.4 g Protein 8.8 g

Cinnamon Almond Flour Bread

Servings: 12

Cooking Time: 35 Minutes

Ingredients:

- 2 cups fine, blanched almond flour
- 2 tbsp coconut flour
- ½ tsp sea salt
- 1 tsp baking soda
- ¼ cup flaxseed meal
- 5 eggs + 1 egg white
- 1 ½ tsp apple cider vinegar
- 2 tbsp maple syrup or honey
- 2–3 tbsp clarified butter (melted)
- 1 tbsp cinnamon + extra for topping

Directions:

1. Preheat your oven to 350 degrees F. Layer an 8x4-inch loaf pan with wax paper.
2. In a bowl, mix coconut flour, baking soda, salt, almond flour, flaxseed meal, and ½ tbsp cinnamon.
3. Beat the egg white and eggs separately then stir in maple syrup, vinegar, and 1 tbsp butter.
4. Stir in coconut flour mixture and combine until smooth.
5. Spread the batter evenly in the loaf pan.

6. Bake the bread for 35 minutes at 350 degrees F.

7. Allow it to cool on a wire rack.

8. Mix 1 tbsp melted butter with ½ tbsp cinnamon and brush this butter over the bread.

9. Serve.

Nutrition Info: Calories Total Fat 5.9 g Saturated Fat 1.5 g Cholesterol 3 mg Sodium 313 mg Total Carbs 8.5 g Fiber 3.2 g Sugar 3.7 g Protein 4.7 g

Nutmeg Gingersnap Cookies

Servings: 8

Cooking Time: 12 Minutes

Ingredients:

- 2 cups almond flour
- ¼ cup butter, unsalted
- 1 cup erythritol
- 1 large egg
- 1 teaspoon vanilla essence
- ¼ teaspoon salt
- 2 teaspoons ground ginger
- ¼ teaspoon ground nutmeg
- ¼ teaspoon ground cloves
- ½ teaspoon cinnamon, ground

Directions:

1. Let the oven preheat at 350 degrees F.
2. Spread the parchment paper on a cookie sheet
3. First, beat the wet ingredients in an electric mixer.
4. Then stir in everything else and mix until smooth.
5. Divide the dough into small cookies on the cookie sheet spoon by spoon.
6. Bake them for 12 mins in the preheated oven.
7. Enjoy.

Nutrition Info: Calories 77. ;Total Fat 7.13 g ;Saturated Fat 4.5 g ;Cholesterol 15 mg ;Sodium 15 mg ;Total Carbs 0.8 g ;Sugar 0.2 g ;Fiber 0.3 g ;Protein 2.3 g

Keto Pignoli Cookies

Servings: 35-40

Cooking Time: 10 – 12 Minutes

Ingredients:

- 2 large eggs
- ¼ teaspoon salt
- 4 cups superfine blanched almond flour (do not use almond meal)
- 2 teaspoons almond extract
- 2 cups granulated erythritol + extra to sprinkle if desired
- 2/3 cup Pignoli nuts (also called as pine nuts)

Directions:

1. Add eggs, salt, almond extract and sweetener into a large mixing bowl.
2. Whisk well with an electric hand mixer for 3 minutes.
3. Beat in the almond flour. Continue beating until dough is formed. If the prepared dough is very dry. Sprinkle a tablespoon of water at a time and mix well each time.
4. Add pignoli nuts into a shallow bowl.
5. Divide the dough into 340 equal portions and shape into balls.
6. Line 2 large cookie sheets with parchment paper.

7. Press the balls (only one side) over the pignoli nuts and place on the cookie sheet, with the nut side facing up. Leave gap between the cookies while placing them on the baking sheet.

8. Bake in a preheated oven at 325° F for about 10 – 12 minutes or until light brown around the edges.

9. Remove from the oven and cool for 3-4 minutes. Remove the cookies carefully with a metal spatula and cool on a wire rack.

10. Sprinkle erythritol if desired.

11. Transfer into an airtight container. Refrigerate until use. These can keep for 7-8 days. If you freeze the cookies These can keep for 6 months.

Nutrition Info: Per Servings: Calories: 80.8 kcal, Fat: 5.4 g, Carbohydrates: 2.8 g, Protein: 2.9 g

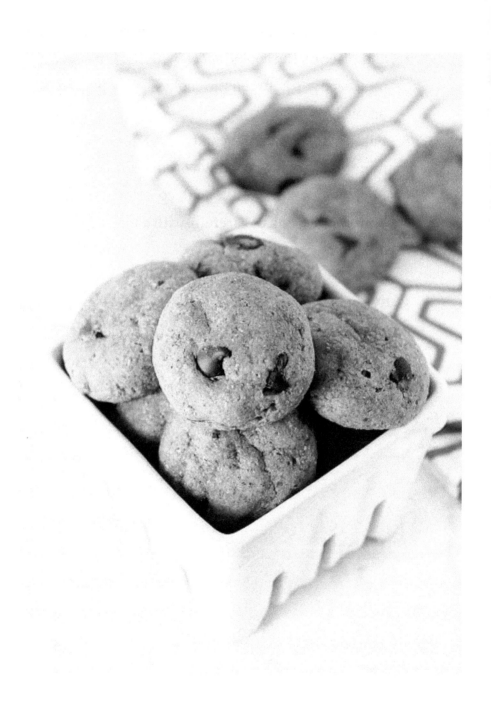

Almond Pumpkin Cookies

Servings: 27

Cooking Time: 25 Minutes

Ingredients:

- 1 egg
- 1 tsp liquid stevia
- 12 tsp pumpkin pie spice
- 12 cup pumpkin puree
- 2 cups almond flour
- 12 tsp baking powder
- 1 tsp vanilla
- 12 cup butter

Directions:

1. Preheat the oven to 300 F 0.
2. Spray a baking tray with cooking spray and set aside.
3. In a large bowl, add all ingredients and mix until well combined.
4. Make cookies from mixture and place onto a prepared baking tray.
5. Bake for 20-2minutes.
6. Remove cookies from oven and set aside to cool completely.
7. Serve and enjoy.

Nutrition Info: Per Servings: Net Carbs: 0.2g; Calories: Total Fat: 7.7g; Saturated Fat: 2.5g Protein: 2.1g; Carbs: 2.2g; Fiber: 1g; Sugar: 0.5g; Fat 87% Protein 12% Carbs 1%

Cream Dipped Cookies

Servings: 8

Cooking Time: 25 Minutes

Ingredients:

- 1 cup almond flour
- ½ cup cacao nibs
- ½ cup coconut flakes, unsweetened
- 1/3 cup erythritol
- ½ cup almond butter
- ¼ cup butter, melted
- 2 large eggs
- Stevia, to taste
- ¼ teaspoon salt
- Glaze:
- ¼ cup heavy whipping cream
- 1/8 teaspoon xanthan gum
- Stevia, to taste
- Optional: ½ teaspoon vanilla essence

Directions:

1. Let your oven preheat at 350 degrees F.
2. Combine all the dry ingredients in a suitably sized bowl.
3. Beat stevia, almond butter, butter, and vanilla essence in the eggs.

4. Stir in the almond flour mixture and whisk well.

5. Make 16 cookies on a cookie sheet by dropping the batter spoon by spoon.

6. Press each cookie to flatten it.

7. Bake them for 25 mins in the preheated oven.

8. During this time, combine the glaze ingredients in a saucepan.

9. Let them cook until the sauce thickens.

10. Once the cookies are done, place them over the wire rack.

11. Pour this cooked glaze over the cookies equally.

12. Allow this glaze to set in 15 minutes.

13. Enjoy.

Nutrition Info: Calories 192 ;Total Fat 17.44 g ;Saturated Fat 11.5 g ;Cholesterol 125 mg ;Sodium 135 mg ;Total Carbs 2.2 g ;Sugar 1.4 g ;Fiber 2.1 g ;Protein 4.7 g

Cinnamon Snickerdoodle Balls

Servings: 8

Cooking Time: 12 Minutes

Ingredients:

- Cookies:
- 2 eggs
- 2 teaspoons vanilla essence
- 1 cup almond butter
- 1/2 cup almond milk
- 1/4 cup coconut oil, solid, at
- 1 1/2 cup monk fruit sweetener
- 1 3/4 cup almond flour
- 1 cup coconut flour
- 1 teaspoon baking soda
- 2 teaspoons tartar cream
- 1/8 teaspoon pink Himalayan salt
- 1 teaspoon cinnamon
- Topping:
- 3 tablespoons monk fruit sweetener
- 1 tablespoon cinnamon

Directions:

1. Let your oven preheat at 350 degrees F.
2. Line a cookie sheet with wax paper.

3. Add the wet ingredients of the cookies to a blender and beat well.

4. Stir in dry mixture and combine them well.

5. Place this batter in the refrigerator for 1minutes to set.

6. Make small balls out of this mixture.

7. Mix cinnamon and monk fruit in a shallow plate.

8. Roll these balls into this mixture to coat well.

9. Bake these balls in a baking sheet for 12 minutes.

10. Serve once cooled.

Nutrition Info: Calories 252 ;Total Fat 17.3 g ;Saturated Fat 5 g ;Cholesterol 141 mg ;Sodium 153 mg ;Total Carbs 7.2 g ;Sugar 0.3 g ;Fiber 1.4 g ;Protein 5.2 g

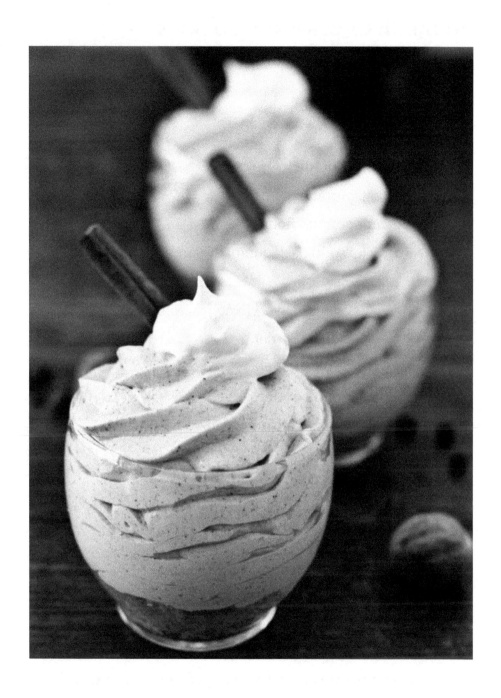

Pumpkin Cheesecake Cookies

Servings: 12

Cooking Time: 20 Minutes

Ingredients:

- For the Pumpkin Cookie
- 6 tbsp butter, softened
- 2 cups almond flour
- 1/3 cup solid pack pumpkin puree
- 1 large egg
- ¾ cup granulated erythritol sweetener
- ½ tsp baking powder
- 1 tsp ground cinnamon
- ¼ tsp ground nutmeg
- 1/8 tsp ground allspice
- Pinch of salt
- For the Cheesecake Filling
- 4 oz cream cheese
- ½ tsp vanilla
- 1 large egg
- 2 tbsp granulated erythritol sweetener

Directions:

1. Preheat your oven at 350 degrees F.
2. Add all the cookie dough ingredients to a suitable bowl and form a smooth dough.

3. Add the dough to a cookie sheet lined with wax paper scoop by scoop.

4. Flatten the scoops of dough with a spoon and make a dent in the center of each cookie.

5. Whisk cream cheese with vanilla, egg, and sweetener in a mixer.

6. Divide this mixture into the center of each cookie.

7. Bake them for 20 minutes until golden brown.

8. Allow them to cool for 10 minutes.

9. Enjoy.

Nutrition Info: Calories 175 Total Fat 16 g Saturated Fat 2.1 g Cholesterol 124 mg Sodium 8 mg Total Carbs 2.8 g Sugar 1.8 g Fiber 0.4 g Protein 9 g

Butter Glazed Cookies

Servings: 40

Cooking Time: 6 Minutes

Ingredients:

- 1/3 cup coconut flour
- 2/3 cup almond flour
- ¼ cup granulated erythritol
- 8 drops stevia
- ½ cup butter, softened
- 1 tsp almond or vanilla extract
- ¼ tsp baking powder
- ¼ tsp xanthan gum (optional)
- For the Glaze:
- ¼ cup coconut butter
- 8 drops stevia

Directions:

1. Preheat your oven to 356 degrees F.
2. Whisk dry ingredients in one bowl and beat butter with stevia and vanilla extract in another.
3. Add dry mixture and mix well until smooth then divide the dough into two pieces.
4. Place each dough piece in between two sheets of wax paper.

5. Spread them into a thick sheet and refrigerate for 10 minutes.

6. Use a cookies cutter to cut small cookies out of both the dough sheets.

7. Place them on a baking sheet lined with wax paper and bake them for 6 minutes.

8. Meanwhile, prepare the glaze by heating coconut butter with stevia in a bowl in the microwave.

9. Pour this glaze over each cookie and allow it to set.

10. Serve.

Nutrition Info: Calories 237 Total Fat 22 g Saturated Fat 9 g Cholesterol 35 mg Sodium mg Total Carbs 5 g Sugar 1 g Fiber 2 g Protein 5 g

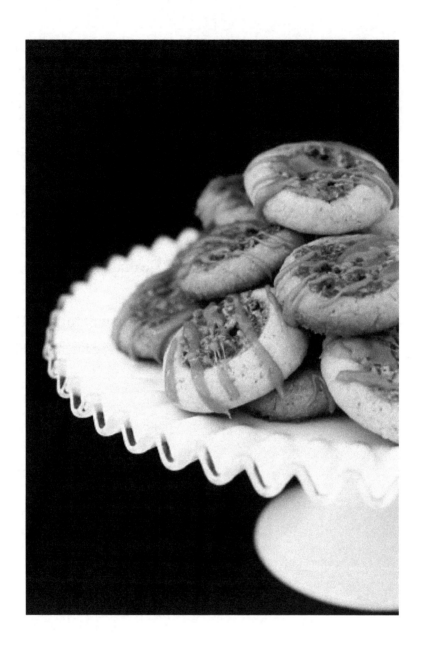

Pecan Pie Cookies

Servings: 23

Cooking Time: 40 Minutes

Ingredients:

- 1 cup almonds
- 1/4 cup chia seeds
- 1/4 cup chocolate chips, unsweetened
- 1 cup pecans, and more for topping
- 1 cup candied pecans, sugar-free
- 1/2 cup erythritol sweetener
- 1 cup almond butter
- 1/4 cup coconut milk

Directions:

1. Place all pecans and almonds in a food processor and pulse for minute or more until crumbled.
2. Add remaining ingredients and blend until thick mixture comes together, add more milk if the mixture is crumbly.
3. Tip the mixture in a large bowl, then shape into 2cookie balls and place on a baking tray, lined with parchment paper.
4. Top cookies with more pecans and chill in the refrigerator for 30 minutes or until firm.
5. Serve straightaway.

Nutrition Info: Calories: 1 Cal, Carbs: 5 g, Fat: 16 g, Protein: 5 g, Fiber: 4 g.

Crunchy Shortbread Cookies

Servings: 6

Cooking Time: 10 Minutes

Ingredients:

- 1 ¼ cup almond flour
- ½ tsp vanilla
- 3 tbsp butter, softened
- ¼ cup Swerve
- Pinch of salt

Directions:

1. Preheat the oven to 350 F 0 C.
2. In a bowl, mix together almond flour, swerve, and salt.
3. Add vanilla and butter and mix until dough is formed.
4. Make cookies from mixture and place on a baking tray.
5. Bake in preheated oven for 10 minutes.
6. Allow to cool completely then serve.

Nutrition Info: Per Servings: Net Carbs: 2.6g; Calories: 185; Total Fat: 14g; Saturated Fat: 4.5g Protein: 5.1g; Carbs: 5.1g; Fiber: 2.5g; Sugar: 0.9g; Fat 84% Protein 11% Carbs 5%

Flax Seed Muffins

Servings: 12

Cooking Time: 21 Minutes

Ingredients:

- 1 Cup of ground golden flax seed
- 4 Large Pastured eggs
- ½ Cup of avocado oil or any type of oil
- ½ Cup of swerve
- ¼ Cup of coconut flour
- 2 Teaspoons of vanilla extract
- 2 Teaspoons of cinnamon
- 1 Teaspoon of lemon juice
- ½ Teaspoon of baking soda
- 1 Pinch of sea salt
- 1 Cup of chopped walnuts

Directions:

1. Preheat your oven to a temperature of about 325 F.
2. If the flaxseed is not ground, grind it with a coffee grinder.
3. Mix the flax seeds with the pastured eggs, the avocado oil, the Swerve, the coconut flour, the vanilla extract, the cinnamon, the lemon juice, the baking soda, the salt and the walnuts with an electric mixer.

4. Prepare a muffin pan of 12 holes and line it with silicone muffin cups or parchment paper cups.

5. Distribute the batter evenly between the muffin cups; then bake it for about 18 to 21 minutes at a temperature of 32F.

6. Serve and enjoy your muffins!

Nutrition Info: Calories: 218;Fat: 20g;Carbohydrates: 6g;Fiber: 3g;Protein: 6.3

Almond Butter Cookies

Servings: 10

Cooking Time: 10 Minutes

Ingredients:

- 1 cup almond flour
- 1 tsp vanilla
- ¼ cup erythritol
- ¼ cup butter softened
- Pinch of salt

Directions:

1. Preheat the oven to 350 F 0 C.
2. Line baking tray with parchment paper and set aside.
3. Add all ingredients into the food processor and process until dough is formed, about 2 minutes.
4. Make cookies from dough and place on a prepared baking tray.
5. Bake in preheated oven for 10 minutes.
6. Remove cookies from oven and allow to cool completely.
7. Serve and enjoy.

Nutrition Info: Per Servings: Net Carbs: 1.3g; Calories: 106; Total Fat: 10.2g; Saturated Fat: 3.3g Protein: 2.5g; Carbs: 2.5g; Fiber: 1.2g; Sugar: 0.5g; Fat % Protein 10% Carbs 4%

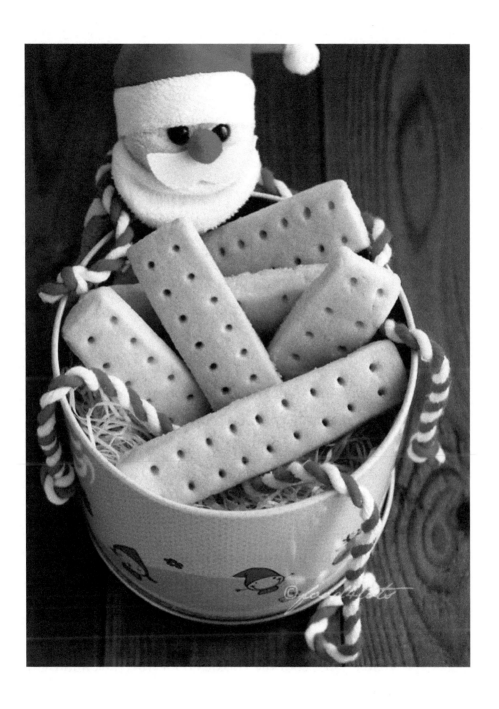

Shortbread Cookies

Servings: 16

Cooking Time: 35 Minutes

Ingredients:

- 2 cups almond flour
- 1/16 teaspoon salt
- 1/3 cup erythritol sweetener
- 1 teaspoon vanilla extract, unsweetened
- 1/2 cup softened butter, unsalted
- 1 egg

Directions:

1. Set oven to 350 degrees F and let preheat.
2. In the meantime, place flour in a large bowl, add salt, sweetener, and vanilla and mix well.
3. Add butter and rub until thoroughly combined.
4. Add egg, mix well and then shape mixture into 16 cookie balls.
5. Place cookie balls on a parchment lined cookie sheet and place into the oven.
6. Bake cookies for 15 to 25 minutes or until edges are nicely brown and cookies are firm.
7. When done, cool the cookies on a wire rack and then serve.

Nutrition Info: Calories: 126 Cal, Carbs: 2 g, Fat: 12 g, Protein: 3 g, Fiber: 1 g.

Sugar-free Sugar

Servings: 24

Cooking Time: 6 Hours 25 Minutes

Ingredients:

- 1 1/4 cups almond flour
- 1/2 tsp. baking powder, gluten-free
- 5 tbsp. butter
- 1/2 cup monk fruit sweetener, granulated
- 1 tsp. vanilla extract, sugar-free
- 1/2 tsp. almond extract
- 4 tbsp. coconut flour
- 1 large egg
- 1/4 tsp. salt

Directions:

1. Place a piece of saran wrap to the side.
2. In a big dish, cream the sweetener, vanilla extract, and butter with an electrical beater until smooth. Add the egg, baking powder, and almond extract until fluffy and light.
3. Stir in the almond flour, salt and coconut flour with a rubber scraper.Transfer the dough to the saran wrap, roll into a large ball and wrap tightly.Refrigerate the wrapped dough for a least 6 hours. Alternatively, it can be left overnight.

4. After the dough is firm, make sure your stove is set at 375 ° Fahrenheit. Use a non-stick baking mat or cover a regular sized cookie sheet with baking paper.Using 2 pieces of baking paper, place the chilled dough in between them and roll to approximately 1/inch thick.

5. Use the size and shape of cookie cutters that you prefer and cut the dough. Transfer the cut cookies to the prepared cookie sheet using a large spatula.

6. Heat in the stove for 10 − 11 minutes until golden. Remove the sheet to the counter. Wait 10 minutes for the cookies to cool before serving.

Nutrition Info: 2 grams ;Net Carbs: 0.8 grams ;Fat: 5 grams ;Calories: 59

Almond Cinnamon Butter Cookies

Servings: 8

Cooking Time: 15 Minutes

Ingredients:

- 1/2 cup butter, softened
- 2 cups blanched almond flour
- 1 egg
- 1/2 cup swerve
- 1 teaspoon vanilla essence
- 1 teaspoon cinnamon ground

Directions:

1. Let your oven preheat at 350 degrees F. Layer a baking sheet with wax paper.
2. Toss almond flour with egg, butter, cinnamon, vanilla and swerve in a bowl.
3. Make 1-inch balls out of it and place them in a baking sheet.
4. Press them into cookies and make a criss-cross pattern over each cookie using a fork.
5. Bake them for 1minutes until golden.
6. Allow them to cool.
7. Serve.

Nutrition Info: Per Servings: Calories 192 Total Fat 17.44 g Saturated Fat 11.5 g Cholesterol 125 mg Total Carbs 2.2 g

Sugar 1.4 g Fiber 2.1 g Sodium 135 mg Potassium 53 mg
Protein 4.7 g

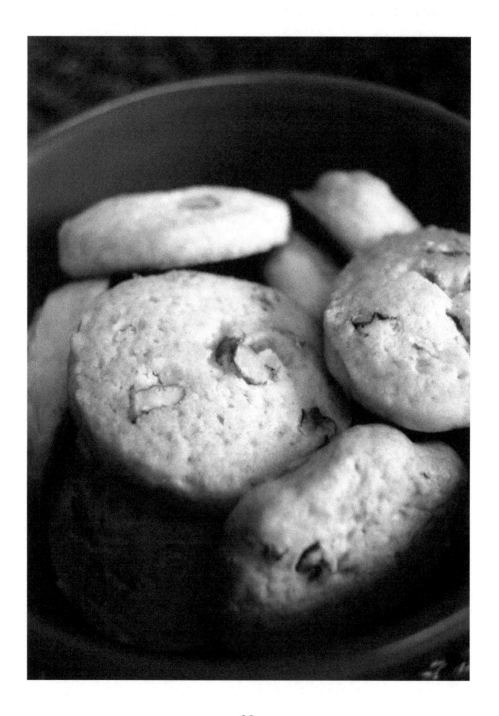

Pecan Cookies

Servings: 16

Cooking Time: 20 Minutes

Ingredients:

- 1 cup pecans
- 13 cup coconut flour
- 1 cup almond flour
- 12 cup butter
- 1 tsp vanilla
- 2 tsp gelatin
- 23 cup Swerve

Directions:

1. Preheat the oven to 350 F 0 C.
2. Spray a baking tray with cooking spray and set aside.
3. Add butter, vanilla, gelatin, swerve, coconut flour, and almond flour into the food processor and process until crumbs form.
4. Add pecans and process until chopped.
5. Make cookies from prepared mixture and place onto a prepared baking tray.
6. Bake in for 20 minutes.
7. Serve and enjoy.

Nutrition Info: Per Servings: Net Carbs: 1.3g; Calories: 146; Total Fat: 14.; Saturated Fat: 4.4g Protein: 2.4g; Carbs: 2.9g; Fiber: 1.6g; Sugar: 0.6g; Fat 91% Protein 6% Carbs 3%

Vanilla Shortbread Cookies

Servings: 6

Cooking Time: 15 Minutes

Ingredients:

- 2 1/2 cups almond flour
- 6 tablespoons butter
- 1/2 cup erythritol
- 1 teaspoon vanilla essence

Directions:

1. Let your oven preheat at 350 degrees F.
2. Spread a parchment paper in a cookie sheet.
3. Beat erythritol in the butter until it turns frothy.
4. Add in flour and vanilla essence while beating the mixture.
5. Divide this batter on a cookie sheet in small cookies.
6. Bake those cookies for 15 mins in the preheated oven at 350 degrees F.
7. Serve and enjoy.

Nutrition Info: Calories 2 ;Total Fat 25.3 g ;Saturated Fat 6.7 g ;Cholesterol 23 mg ;Sodium 74 mg ;Total Carbs 9.6 g ;Sugar 0.1 g ;Fiber 3.8 g ;Protein 7.6 g

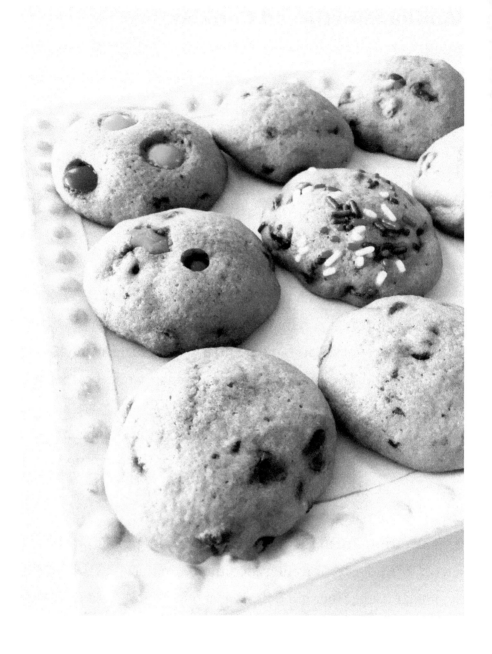

Fluffy Cookies

Servings: 8

Cooking Time: 15 Minutes

Ingredients:

- 2 eggs
- ½ tsp baking powder
- 5 tbsp butter, melted
- 13 cup sour cream
- 13 cup mozzarella cheese, shredded
- 1 ¼ cup almond flour
- ½ tsp salt

Directions:

1. Preheat the oven to 400 F 200 C.
2. Spray muffin pan with cooking spray and set aside.
3. Add all ingredients into a large bowl and mix well using a hand mixer.
4. Spoon batter into the muffin tray, filling the muffin cups around 23.
5. Bake in preheated oven for 12-1minutes.
6. Remove cookies from oven and let it cool for 5 minutes.
7. Serve and enjoy.

Nutrition Info: Per Servings: Net Carbs: 2.5g; Calories: 204 Total Fat: 19.3g; Saturated Fat: 6.9g Protein: 5.; Carbs: 4.4g; Fiber: 1.9g; Sugar: 0.7g; Fat 85% Protein 11% Carbs 4%

Cocoa Keto Cookies

Servings: 11

Cooking Time: 15 Minutes

Ingredients:

- ½ Cup of Swerve confectioner
- ½ Cup of Unsweetened Cocoa Powder
- 4 Tablespoons of almond butter
- 2 Large Eggs
- 1 Teaspoon of vanilla extract
- 1 Cup of Almond Flour
- 1 Teaspoon of baking powder
- 1 Pinch of Pink Salt

Directions:

1. Combine the cocoa powder with the swerve in a large mixing bowl; then add then add the melted butter to the mixture and combine all together with the help of a hand mixer.
2. Once your ingredients are very well combined, add the eggs, the vanilla, and the baking powder and mix again.
3. Add in the almond flour and mix again; the batter should be thick.
4. Form cookies from the dough and arrange it over a baking sheet.

5. Bake your cookies for about 13 to 14 minutes at a temperature if about 3 F.
6. Serve and enjoy your cookies or store them in a clean container to serve whenever you want!

Nutrition Info: Calories: 168;Fat: 14 g;Carbohydrates: 2.5g;Fiber: 1g;Protein: 4

Cocoa Muffins

Servings: 12

Cooking Time: 20 Minutes

Ingredients:

- 1 ¼ Cups of Almond Flour
- ½ Cup of cocoa powder, unsweetened Cocoa Powder
- ½ cup of Erythritol
- 1 and ½ Teaspoons of Baking Powder
- 1 teaspoon of pure Vanilla Extract
- 3 Large eggs
- 2/3 Cup of heavy Cream
- 3 Ounces of melted almond butter
- ½ Cup of Chocolate Chips; Sugar-Free

Directions:

1. Preheat your oven to a temperature of about 350 F.
2. In a large bowl, combine the almond flour with the cocoa powder, the erythritol and the baking powder and mix very well
3. Add in the vanilla extract, the eggs, and the heavy cream and mix very well.
4. Add in the melted coconut oil and mix again
5. Add in the sugar-free chocolate chips to your ingredients and stir very well.
6. Line a muffin tray with cupcake papers

7. Spoon your prepared mixture into the 12 holes of a standard muffin tray or any muffin tray you have
8. Bake your muffins for about 20 minutes
9. Remove the muffins from the oven and let cool for 5 minutes
10. Serve and enjoy your delicious muffins!

Nutrition Info: Calories: 304;Fat: 23 g;Carbohydrates: 9g;Fiber: 2g;Protein: 7

Macadamia Nut Cookies

Servings: 12

Cooking Time: 15 Minutes

Ingredients:

- ½ cup butter, melted
- 2 tbsp almond butter
- 1 egg
- 1 ½ cup almond flour
- 2 tbsp unsweetened cocoa powder
- ½ cup granulated erythritol sweetener
- 1 tsp vanilla extract
- ½ tsp baking soda
- ¼ cup chopped macadamia nuts
- Pinch of salt

Directions:

1. Preheat your oven to 350 degrees F.
2. Whisk all the ingredients well in a bowl with a fork until smooth.
3. Layer a cookie sheet with wax paper and drop the dough onto it scoop by scoop.
4. Flatten each scoop into 1.5-inch wide round.
5. Bake them for 1minutes then allow them to cool.
6. Enjoy.

Nutrition Info: Calories 114 Total Fat 9.6 g Saturated Fat 4.5 g Cholesterol 10 mg Sodium 155 mg Total Carbs 3.1 g Sugar 1.4 g Fiber 1.5 g Protein 3.5 g

Oreo Cookies

Servings: 50 - 60

Cooking Time: 12-13 Minutes

Ingredients:

- For cookies (dry ingredients):
- 4 ½ cups almond or hazelnut flour
- 8 tablespoons cocoa powder
- 1 teaspoon xanthan gum
- 6 tablespoons coconut flour
- 2 teaspoons baking powder
- ½ teaspoon salt
- For cookies (wet ingredients):
- 1 cup butter, softened
- 2 eggs
- 1 cup Swerve sweetener
- 2 teaspoons vanilla extract
- For cream filling:
- 8 ounces cream cheese, softened
- 1 teaspoons vanilla extract
- 4 tablespoons butter
- 1 cup powdered Swerve

Directions:

1. Line 2 large cookie sheets with parchment paper.

2. Add almond flour, cocoa, coconut flour, xanthan gum, salt and baking powder into a large bowl. Mix well.

3. Add butter and sweetener into a mixing bowl. Beat with an electric mixer at medium-high speed until butter blend turns creamy.

4. Add eggs and vanilla extract and beat well.

5. Lower the speed to low speed. Add the mixture of dry ingredients and beat until dough is formed.

6. Place a sheet of parchment paper or baking paper on your countertop. Place the dough on the center of the sheet. Place another sheet on top of the dough.

7. Roll with a rolling pin until the dough is about 1/8 inch thick.

8. Take a cookie cutter of about 1 ½ inches diameter and cut the cookies.

9. Place the cookies on the baking sheet. Leave some gap between the cookies.

10. Collect the scrap dough (after cutting into cookies) and reshape into a ball of dough.

11. Repeat steps 6 – 10 (1 – 2 times) and make more cookies. You should have at least 100 cookies.

12. Bake in a preheated oven at 350° F for about 10 – 13 minutes or until light golden brown. Bake in batches.

13. Remove the baking sheet from the oven and let cookies cool on the baking sheet completely.

14. Meanwhile, make the filling as follows: Add cream cheese and butter into a food processor bowl.
15. Process until creamy. Add vanilla and Swerve and pulse until well combined.
16. Spread filling on half the cookies. Complete the sandwich cookies by covering with the remaining cookies.
17. Transfer into an airtight container. These can keep for 7 – 8 days in the refrigerator. If you freeze the cookies they can keep for 3 months.

Nutrition Info: per Servings: Calories: 123.9 kcal, Fat: 11.6 g, Carbohydrates: 3.2 g, Protein: 3 g

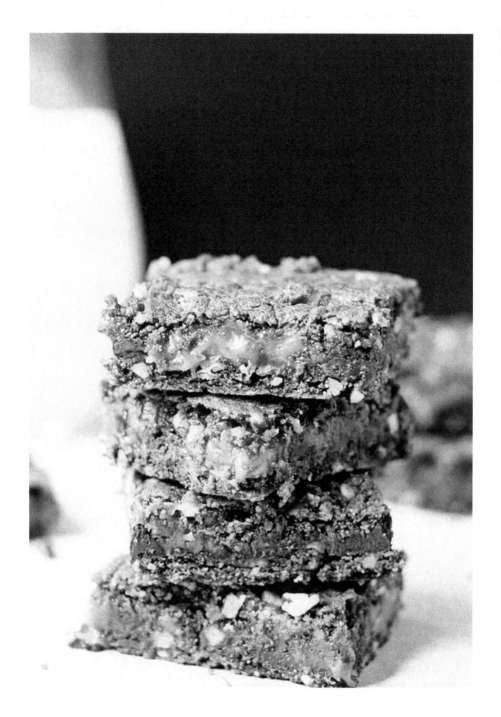

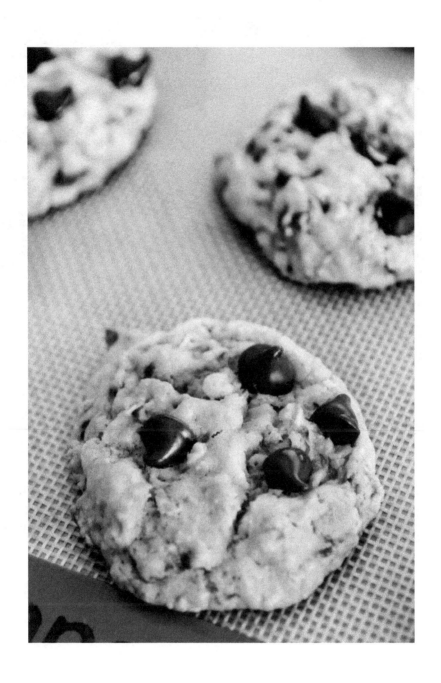

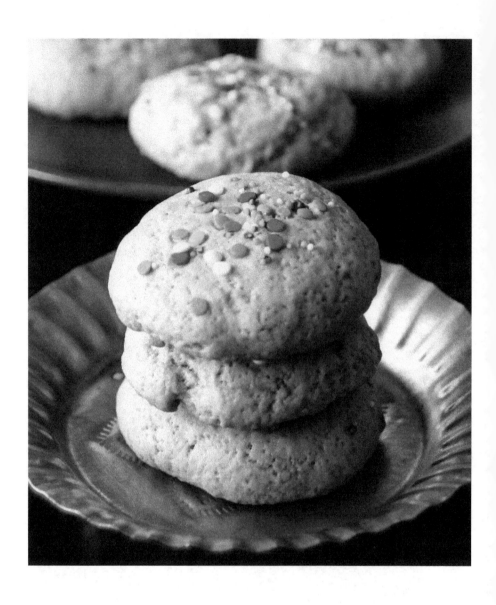